YOUR KNOWLEDGE HAS VALUE

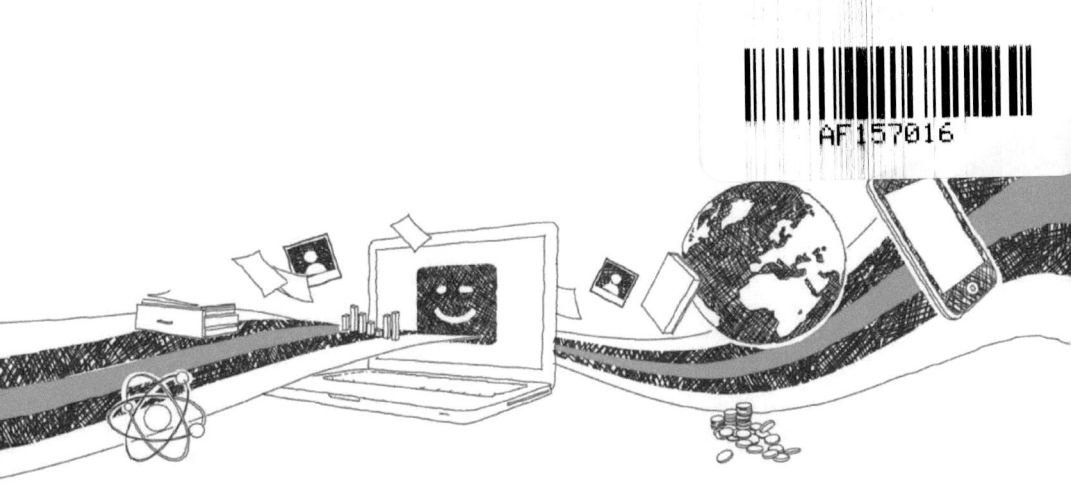
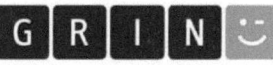

Bibliographic information published by the German National Library:

The German National Library lists this publication in the National Bibliography; detailed bibliographic data are available on the Internet at http://dnb.dnb.de .

Imprint:

Copyright © 2016 GRIN Verlag, Open Publishing GmbH
Print and binding: Books on Demand GmbH, Norderstedt Germany
ISBN: 9783668308459

This book at GRIN:

http://www.grin.com/en/e-book/340946/growth-retardation-in-children-with-atopic-dermatitis

Anjum Hashmi, Fayaz Mamluh Alazmi, Shahid Hashmi

Growth retardation in children with Atopic Dermatitis

GRIN Publishing

GRIN - Your knowledge has value

Since its foundation in 1998, GRIN has specialized in publishing academic texts by students, college teachers and other academics as e-book and printed book. The website www.grin.com is an ideal platform for presenting term papers, final papers, scientific essays, dissertations and specialist books.

Visit us on the internet:

http://www.grin.com/

http://www.facebook.com/grincom

http://www.twitter.com/grin_com

ASSOCIATION OF GROWTH RETARDATION IN CHILDREN WITH ATOPIC DERMATITIS

TABLE OF CONTENTS

LIST OF TABLES iii
ABSTRACT 1
INTRODUCTION 2
REVIEW OF LITERATURE 3
    ATOPIC DERMATITIS 3
    EPIDEMIOLOGY 3
    ETIOLOGY AND PATHOGENESIS 3
    EXACERBATING FACTORS FOR ATOPIC DERMATITIS 8
    HISTOPATHOLOGY OF ATOPIC DERMATITIS 11
    DIAGNOSIS OF ATOPIC DERMATITIS 12
    DIFFERENTIAL DIAGNOSIS[18] OF ATOPIC DERMATITIS 12
    COMPLICATIONS OF ATOPIC DERMATITIS 14
    GROWTH IMPAIRMENT 14
    ASSESSMENT OF GROWTH 20
OBJECTIVE 21
OPERATIONAL DEFINITIONS 21
    ATOPIC DERMATITIS 21
    SEVERITY 21
    GROWTH RETARDATION 21
MATERIAL AND METHODS 22
    SETTING 22
    DURATION OF STUDY 22
    SAMPLE SIZE 22
    SAMPLING TECHNIQUE 22
    STUDY DESIGN 22
    SAMPLE SELECTION 22
    DATA ANALYSIS 23
FREQUENCY OF GROWTH RETARDATION IN CHILDREN WITH MODERATE TO
SEVERE ATOPIC DERMATITIS 24
RESULTS 25
DISCUSSION 33
    CONCLUSION 34
REFERENCES 35
Annexure 1 42
Annexure 2 43

LIST OF TABLES

i. Table 1: Demographic data

LIST OF FIGURES

i.   Figure 1: Age distribution

ii.   Figure 2: Sex distribution

iii   Figure 3: Height distribution

iv   Figure 4: Weight distribution

v   Figure 5: Comparison of normal and growth retarded children

vi Figure 6: Comparison of growth retardation between

                         moderate and severe atopic dermatitis

vii Figure 7: Comparison of growth retardation in male and female

LIST OF ABBREVIATIONS

AD	Atopic dermatitis
IL	Interleukin
FLG	Filaggrin
EFA's	Essential fatty acids
GH	Growth hormone
IGF-1	Insulin like growth factor-1
IGF-2	Insulin like growth factor-2
GHRH	Growth hormone releasing hormone
ACTH	Adrenocorticotrophic hormone
FGF21	Fibroblast growth factor 21
PGE2	Prostaglandin E2
PTH	Parathyroid hormone
$1\alpha, 25(OH)_2 D_3$	1α, 25-dihydroxyvitamin D_3
NCHS	National Centre of Health Statistics
CDC	Centers for Disease Control and Prevention

ABSTRACT

Introduction: Atopic dermatitis (AD) is a chronic inflammatory skin disorder, associated with significant morbidity. One of the complications associated with AD is growth retardation. **Objective:** The objective of this study was to determine the frequency of growth retardation in children with moderate to severe atopic dermatitis.

Study Design: Cross sectional survey

Setting: WAPDA Hospital, Lahore, a 300 bedded facility

Method: Forty children with AD fulfilling the inclusion criteria were entered in the study. Height was recorded, in centimeters, using infantometer in children ≤ 3 years and with stadiometer in patients > 3 years. Weight was taken, in kilograms, using Tanita baby scale for children ≤ 3 years and Bath room weighing scale for patients > 3 years. Growth charts were selected according to age and gender of patients. Measurements and percentile ranks of patients were noted on appropriate charts, if they were below 3rd percentile on any of these charts, then child was taken as suffering from growth retardation. **Results:** Twenty five (62.5%) children had normal growth while 15 (37.5%) patients had growth retardation. Among these 15 retarded children, 9 (22.5%) were suffering from moderate disease and 6 (15%) had severe disease. Out of total 40 patients, 11 had severe disease and 6 (54.54%) of them were suffering from growth retardation, while 29 had moderate disease and 9 (31.03%) of them showed impaired growth. Nine (22.5%) of patients with growth impairment were female and 6 (15%) were male.

Conclusion: These results show growth retardation in children with atopic dermatitis. The frequency of growth impairment was relatively more in severe disease and among girls, as depicted by growth charts.

Keywords: Atopic dermatitis; Growth retardation; Growth chart; Lahore; Pakistan

INTRODUCTION

AD is a chronic, relapsing, inflammatory skin disorder which is characterized by itchy papules, vesicles, excoriations and lichenification.[1] It is often associated with personal or family history of other atopic conditions such as asthma, allergic rhinitis or hay fever.[2] Diagnosis is made clinically on the basis of history and examination.[3] Genetic, environmental, skin barrier defects and immunological factors are involved in its pathogenesis.[4]

The prevalence of AD varies greatly in children, with less than 2% in China and Iran and upto 20% in northern and western Europe, Australia and the United States.[5] AD is the most common type of eczema seen in children in Pakistan.[6] About 70% cases of atopic dermatitis begin in children under 5 years.[7]

AD has profound impact on quality of life and causes significant morbidity. One of the complications associated with AD is growth impairment in affected children.[8] In majority of cases aetiology of growth retardation is not clear, but atopy related imbalance in local growth factors like prostaglandin E2 (which is a substance important for both allergic reactions and bone metabolism), disturbed sleep and failure of nocturnal growth hormone release during stage 4 sleep can be postulated to impair growth in atopic children.[9,10] Factors like topical, oral or inhaled steroids, co-existing asthma, unnecessary dietary restrictions and vitamin D deficiency may contribute.[11,12]

Growth retardation can be directly related to disease as it was seen in patients of AD before advent of corticosteroids.[12] Association of allergic disorders with growth impairment, had been first described by Cohen et al in 1940.[8] Since that time various studies have been carried out to support the fact. Massarano et al[13] studied 68 children, aged 2-12 years, with AD at University of Manchester and found that mean height of 41 patients with less than 50% of surface area affected was normal while 27 children with more than 50% area affected were significantly shorter. Similarly, Dhar et al[12] studied growth in 100 Indian children with moderate to severe AD and found that 42% of children had weight below 3rd percentile for age and 34% had height below 3rd percentile for age.

The importance of regular growth monitoring in children with AD needs to be emphasized, as if modifiable factors causing growth impairment are taken care of, it will have an impact on overall patient management. There is lack of data on growth pattern of Pakistani children afflicted with AD.

REVIEW OF LITERATURE

ATOPIC DERMATITIS

Definition

AD is a chronic, relapsing inflammatory skin disorder, characterized by itchy skin lesions and personal or family history of other atopic diseases, including asthma and allergic rhinitis.[1]

Atopy

In 1923, Coca and Cooke introduced the term 'atopy' to describe the clinical presentation of type 1 hypersenstivity reactions that exhibit a strong familial predisposition and are associated with elevated IgE levels. The common clinical manifestations of atopy include AD, asthma, hay fever, urticaria and food allergies.[1, 14]

EPIDEMIOLOGY

AD is a common disease, affecting 15 to 30% of children and 2 to 10% of adults. Different studies demonstrate a definite trend towards the increase in AD cases, particularly in industrialized nations over the past few decades.[15, 16] The prevalence of AD varies greatly, with less than 2% in China and Iran and upto 20% in northern and western Europe, Australia and the United States.[5] AD is the most common type of eczema seen in children in Pakistan.[6]

ETIOLOGY AND PATHOGENESIS

A complex interaction of genetic and environmental factors are believed to induce immunological changes, that result in inflammation of skin.[17]

Genetic Factors

Atopic dermatitis is a complex genetic disease that arises from gene–gene and gene–environment interactions. The disease results from abnormalities in genes encoding epidermal structural proteins or major elements of the immune system. AD

3

runs in families, with a strong maternal influence. The concordance rate for AD is higher among monozygotic twins than the dizygotic twins.[18] The prevalence of AD in children is about 50% when one parent has AD, while it may be as high as about 80% when both parents have the disease.[19] A number of genes related to AD have been identified, including genes on chromosomes 1q21, 3p26, 5q31-33, 13q21, 16p11.2-12, 17q11, 17q25 and 20p.[15] Genetic aberrations may result in predominance of Th2 cytokines, increase IgE synthesis, defective epidermal barrier proteins or imbalance between proteases versus protease inhibitors activity, contributing to inflammation.[15, 18]

Immunologic Abnormalities

In response to various allergens, AD patients are genetically prone to produce high levels of IgE.[20] The major disturbance in immune regulatory system that results in this IgE production appears to be the differentiating pathway of helper T cells towards Th2 type cells. The precursor Th0 cells have the potential to differentiate into either Th1 or Th2 type cells, depending upon the signal they receive during interaction with dendritic antigen presenting cells. Th1 cells help in cell mediated immunity; while Th2 cells help B cell function and results in antibody mediated immunity.[1] Epidermal-barrier dysfunction is a prerequisite for the penetration of high-molecular-weight allergens in pollens, house-dust-mite products and microbes. Langerhans' cells are activated on binding of allergens by means of specific IgE receptors and present antigen to Th0 cells. There is the genetic predisposition of atopics to demonstrate predominance of Th2 cells activity over Th1 cells, leading to releases of interleukin-3 (IL-3), IL-4, IL-5, IL-10 and IL-13, which produce eosinophilia in tissue and peripheral blood and increased IgE production, resulting in inflammatory response.[15, 21, 22]

Prostaglandin E2 (PGE2) concentration is also increased in atopics, which also directs differentiation into Th2 type cells. Tissue specificity of the Th2 cell response is explained by cutaneous lymphocyte antigen expression on circulating T cells that specifically home to the skin[17].

Chronic AD lesions principally have a Th1 response with the cytokines IL-12 and interferon-γ playing a dominant role.[17]

Defective Skin Barrier Function

As a part of innate immune system of body, skin is the first line of defense. In AD this barrier function of skin is disrupted through the following:

- Loss of function mutation of epidermal barrier protein, filaggrin

- Reduced ceramide level

- Increased level of endogenous enzymes in skin

- Down regulation of antimicrobial peptides

This impaired barrier function of atopic skin allows greater absorption of allergens, triggering the release of pro-inflammatory mediators.[17, 18, 23]

Loss of Function Mutation of Filaggrin

AD shows genetic linkage to Chromosome 1q21. This region contains the epidermal differentiation complex, which consists of genes that form essential components of epidermal surface and filaggrin (FLG) is one of these. Loss of function mutations of FLG have been identified in AD, which results in defective skin barrier in these patients.[24-28]

Profilaggrin is found in the keratohyalin granules in the stratum granulosum. It is dephosphorylated and proteolytically cleaved to FLG during terminal differentiation of the granular cells. FLG then aggregates keratin filaments, which collapse the granular cells into anuclear squames. The cytoskeleton is then crosslinked by trans-glutaminases to form the cornified cell envelope of the stratum corneum, which is the outer most barrier of skin. Moreover, breakdown products of FLG contribute to the water-binding capacity of the stratum corneum.[24-28]

Reduced Ceramide Level

Stratum corneum lipids are an important determinant for both water retaining and permeability-barrier function in the stratum corneum. Abnormalities in lipid metabolism with reduced synthesis of ceramide may lead to decreased water-binding capacity of skin. Essential fatty acids (EFA's), such as linoleic and linolenic acid, are important components of the epidermal barrier. In atopic dermatitis, Δ^6-desaturase activity is deficient, which leads to decreased linoleic and linolenic acid metabolites. Loss of EFA's results in increased transepidermal water loss and subsequent xerosis. Dryness causes microfissures on the skin surface that promotes entry of irritants, allergens and microbes.[22, 29]

Increased Levels of Endogenous Enzymes in Skin

There are increased levels of endogenous protease enzymes in stratum corneum of AD patients, which break down cellular adhesions, leading to epidermal barrier dysfunction.[30]

Down Regulation of Antimicrobial Peptides

Skin, the first line of defense of the innate immune system, constantly challenged by microbes, have a variety of sensing structures, which include the toll-like receptors, that bind to bacterial, fungal or viral structures and activates epithelial cells to produce antimicrobial peptides known as defensins, cathelicidins, dermicidin and sphingosine. In the case of infection or injury, antimicrobial peptide expression in the skin is upregulated due to increased synthesis by keratinocytes and deposition from degranulation of recruited neutrophils. The inflammatory cytokines, IL-4, IL-10 and IL-13 down regulates these antimicrobial peptides in the skin of patients with AD, resulting in decreased resistance to bacterial, viral and fungal infections.[31-34]

Autoimmunity in Atopic Dermatitis

Patients with atopic dermatitis often have elevated serum IgE levels and sensitization against a variety of environmental allergens, but there is also evidence that exacerbation of the disease occurs in the absence of exposure to external allergens. The IgE antibodies against keratinocytes and endothelial cells are also found in serum of patients with severe AD. These intracellular proteins, which are released as a result of scratching could mimic microbial structures and induce IgE mediated immune response against self proteins, resulting in inflammation.[15]

Abnormalities in Sweating

Sweating is an important trigger of pruritus in AD. This may be due to neuropeptides released in neurogenic control of sweating and IgE mediated allergic reaction to components of sweat. There is altered response to neurogenic stimuli in atopics and increased number of nerve fibers has been found around the sweat glands in their skin.[1]

Abnormal Vascular Reactivity

The small blood vessels in atopics show abnormal vascular reactivity and vasoconstriction responses as:[1]

- White dermographism (Pallor of skin after stroking)

- Delayed blanch phenomenon with acetylcholine

- Marked vasoconstriction on cold exposure and low finger temperature

- Abnormal response to histamine

- White reaction to nicotinic acid esters

Hygiene Hypothesis

AD is a fairly common problem, which in the past half century, has become more prevalent. This increase in atopic diseases has been rationalized by a "hygiene hypothesis," which attributes the propensity towards the atopy associated diseases due to reduced microbial exposure in early life, especially in developed countries. Early life exposure to environmental microbes may cause maturation of the immune system so that dysregulation associated with production of IgE antibody does not occur and this could explain the difference between the western and the developing world regarding the incidence of atopic dermatitis.[35-38]

EXACTERBATING FACTORS FOR ATOPIC DERMATITIS

1. Irritants and Contactants

The skin of patients with AD is very sensitive and vulnerable to irritants. Hot water, soaps, toiletries containing alcohol, astringents, or fragrances, cigarette smoke exposure, enzyme rich laundry detergents, disinfectants, clothing made with synthetic fibers or wool, and juice from fresh fruits such as tomatoes, strawberries and occupational irritants may trigger the itch-scratch cycle.[1,14,22]

2. Airborne Allergens

House dust mite, pollens, moulds, animal dander can aggravate atopic dermatitis.[1]

3. Foods

Dairy products, beef, eggs, chicken, fish, wheat, citrus fruits, food additives, chocolate and nuts, vasodilatory agents, such as alcohol, spices, and hot drinks, histamine-containing foods such as cheese, very ripe vegetables as tomatoes and red wines are common food allergens.[1,14]

4. Microorganisms

Staphylococcus aureus can aggravate AD, and there is usually its overpopulation in atopic patients. The organism is able to induce formation of IgE antibodies and superantigen reactions. Anti staphylococcal therapy can improve AD. In head and neck dermatitis, IgE antibodies to Malassezia furfur can sometimes be demonstrated.[1]

5. Hormones

Exacerbations and remissions in pregnancy, menopause, menses has been noted.[22]

6. Stress

Situations of anxiety, depression, family or work maladaptation may prolong AD and in such situations, neuropeptides are released which exacerbate itching.[22]

7. Climate

Most patients with AD are aware of seasonal variations; disease may improve in summer and worsen in winter. However, heat and exercise induced sweating can trigger AD at anytime of the year.[1,22]

MECHANISM OF PRURITUS

The most disturbing symptom of AD is pruritus, which impairs patient's quality of life. Atopics have an inherently lowered threshold for itching and perceive light mechanical stimuli as itch and not as touch, a phenomenon called allokinesis. Cutaneous free nerve endings in patients with AD appear to be structurally normal, but the density and diameter has been found to be much higher than in normal controls.[22] The effects of therapeutic agents on itching also help us understanding the mediators of pruritus, as the lack of effect of antihistamine argues against the role of histamine, while effectiveness of ciclosporin, capsaicin, opioid antagonist indicate the role of cytokines, neuropeptides and opioids in itching related to AD respectively. Proteases, kinins, and acetylcholine also play a part in pruritus.[1, 39]

Several stimuli are known to trigger the pruritus of AD, common triggers that induce itching in these patients include heat, sweating, wool, xerosis, irritants as soaps, detergents, disinfectants, contact with certain foods, occupational chemicals, emotional stress, alcohol, upper respiratory infections, aeroallergens, cutaneous microbial infections and hormones.[14]

CLINICAL FEATURES

The diagnosis of AD is made clinically on the basis of history and examination. The UK refinement of Hanifin and Rajka's diagnostic criteria is usually applied for diagnosing patients. According to this criteria the child must have:[1]

- an itchy skin condition (or parental report of scratching or rubbing in a child) Plus 3 or more of following:

- Onset below 2 years (not used if child is under 4 years)

- History of skin crease involvement (and/or cheeks in children under 10 years)

- History of generally dry skin

- Personal history of other atopic disease (or history of any atopic disease in a first degree relative in children under 4 years)

- Visible flexural dermatitis (or dermatitis of cheeks/ forehead and outer limbs in children under 4 years)

9

In addition to these diagnostic points, the patients with atopic dermatitis may have following clinical features:[19]

- Anterior subcapsular cataract

- Dennie-Morgan infraorbital fold

- Keratoconus

- Orbital darkening

- Recurrent conjunctivitis

- Cheilitis

- Facial pallor or facial erythema

- Ichthyosis

- Palmar hyperlinearity

- Keratosis pilaris

- Itch when sweating

- Nipple eczema

- Perifollicular accentuation

- Pityriasis alba

- Tendency toward cutaneous infections (especially Staphylococcus aureus and herpes simplex) or impaired-cell mediated immunity

- Tendency toward nonspecific hand or foot dermatitis

- White dermatographism or delayed blanch to cholinergic agents

- Food intolerance

- Intolerance to wool and lipid solvents

Approximately 45 percent of cases of AD begin within the first 6 months of life, 60 percent develop their disease during the first year and 85% begin before 5 years of age.[15]

There are three phases of AD according to age of onset[1]:

1. Infantile phase

2. Childhood phase

3. Adult phase

1. Infantile Atopic Dermatitis

Atopic dermatitis develops from 2 months to 2 years of age.[19] Eruption is more acute and usually starts on face and later on extensor surfaces are involved, as child begins to crawl. The diaper area is usually spared.[1]

2. Childhood Atopic Dermatitis

AD develops from 2 to 10 years of age.[19] The most common sites involved are the antecubital fossae, popliteal fossae, wrists, ankles, and sides of neck.[1]

3. Adult Atopic Dermatitis

The clinical picture of AD in adults is similar to childhood phase, with lichenification, especially of flexural surfaces and hands. In young atopic women, localized patches of eczema may involve the nipples.[1]

Pruritus is the hallmark of the disease in all stages. AD is "the itch that rashes". Lesions of AD may be acute, subacute or chronic. In acute eczema, erythematous papules, plaques, vesicles, serous exudation and excoriations are present. Subacute eczema is characterized by scaly, erythematous, excoriated papules and plaques, while in chronic dermatitis lichenified plaques forms.[14]

HISTOPATHOLOGY OF ATOPIC DERMATITIS

The histopathology shows non specific changes of hyperkeratosis, acanthosis, spongiosis, dermal oedema and infiltration with lymphocytes, histiocytes, plasma cells and eosinophils.[1]

DIAGNOSIS OF ATOPIC DERMATITIS

The diagnosis of AD is made clinically; skin biopsy and other tests are of little value in this regard. Skin-prick, radioallergosorbent tests and serum IgE levels may be useful for assessing the contribution of foods and environmental allergens to disease expression in children with severe disease. Serum IgE levels are normal in about 20 percent of atopic patients. Patch test may be helpful in excluding superimposed allergic contact dermatitis.[1]

If immunodeficiency is suspected in a child, then immunoglobulin and complement levels & functions, white blood cells, platelets, T lymphocytes, B lymphocytes and phagocyte cells counts & functions should be assessed.[1]

DIFFERENTIAL DIAGNOSIS[18] OF ATOPIC DERMATITIS

Most likely

- Contact dermatitis

- Seborrheic dermatitis

- Scabies

- Psoriasis

- Ichthyosis vulgaris

- Keratosis pilaris

- Dermatophytosis

- Impetigo

- Drug reaction

- Pityriasis alba

- Nummular eczema

Less common/Rare (Predominantly in infants/children)

Metabolic/Nutritional

- Zinc deficiency

- Phenylketonuria

Primary immunodeficiency disorders

- Severe combined immunodeficiency

- DisGeorge syndrome

- Hypogammaglobulinemia

- Agammaglobulinemia

- Wiskott-Aldrich syndrome

- Ataxia talengiectasia

Genetic syndromes

- Netherton syndrome

- Hurler syndrome

Others

- Neonatal lupus erythematosus

- Langerhans cell histiocytosis

Less common/Rare (Predominantly in adolescents and adults)

- Cutaneous T cell lymphoma

- Human immunodeficiency virus associated dermatoses

- Lupus erythematosus

- Dermatomyositis

- Graft versus host disease

- Pemphigus foliaceus

- Dermatitis herpetiformis

COMPLICATIONS OF ATOPIC DERMATITIS

Ocular Complications

Eyelid dermatitis, chronic blepharitis, keratoconjuctivitis, uveitis, keratoconus, subcapsular cataract, corneal scarring and retinal detachment are the ocular complications seen in these patients.[40-43]

Infections

AD can be complicated by recurrent viral infections due to defective local T cell function. The most serious is herpes simplex, resulting in eczema herpeticum. Multiple umblicated vesiculopustular lesions forms.[44, 45] In head and neck dermatitis, IgE antibodies to Malassezia furfur can sometimes be demonstrated.[46,47] Staphylococcus aureus aggravates AD, and there is usually its overpopulation in atopic individuals. The organism is able to induce formation of IgE antibodies and superantigen reactions.[48, 49]

Exfoliative Dermatitis

AD may be complicated by exfoliative dermatitis, which is characterized by generalized erythema, scaling, crusting, weeping and constitutional symptoms. It is usually due to superimposed Staphylococcus aureus or herpes simplex infection.[18]

Psychosocial Effects

AD has a significant affect on quality of life secondary to stigmatization of the condition, psychological stress, lack of sleep secondary to pruritus and pain and effects on social and financial well being.[1]

GROWTH IMPAIRMENT

AD can be complicated by growth retardation in affected children, therefore regular growth assessment is an integral part of child care.[1]

Physiology of Growth

Growth is a dynamic and complex physiological process that starts with the fertilization of the ovum and is completed with the fusion of epiphyses and metastases of the long bones, marking the completion of adolescence. Growth

14

occurs in phases, which are influenced mainly by genetic factors, thyroid hormone, cortisol, growth hormone (GH), insulin like growth factor-1(IGF-1), nutritional status and vitamin D.[50]

There are 4 phases of human growth: [50]

Fetal Phase

It is dependent on placental nutritional supply, which in turn affects fetal growth factors, as insulin like growth factor-2 (IGF-2), human placental lactogen and insulin. Intrauterine growth retardation can result in short stature.[50, 51]

Infantile Phase

It is influenced by nutrition and normal thyroid function.[50]

Childhood Phase

Growth hormone secretion from pituitary gland is the main determinant of child's rate of growth, which mediates its effect by producing IGF-1 at epiphyses of bone. Along with this, good nutrition, thyroid hormone, vitamin D and steroids also affect growth.[50]

Pubertal phase

Sex hormones, mainly testosterone and oestradiol, play an important role in GH secretion and growth at puberty.[50]

CAUSES OF GROWTH RETARDATION52[, 53, 54]

Non-Organic/ Environmental

- Poor nutrition

- Psychosocial problems

- Neglect or child abuse[55]

Organic

- Impaired suck/swallow (cleft palate, cleft lip)

- Chronic diseases (Crohn´s disease, cystic fibrosis, chronic renal failure, congenital heart disease, thyrotoxicosis, liver disease, severe asthma)

- Malabsorption (Celiac disease, cystic fibrosis, cow's milk protein intolerance, short gut syndrome)

- Chromosomal disorders e.g. Down's syndrome

- Intrauterine growth retardation, prematurity

- Congenital infections

- Chronic infections e.g. tuberculosis, HIV,[56,57] parasitic infestation

- Metabolic disorder (Thyrotoxicosis, congenital hypothyroidism, growth hormone deficiency, diabetes insipidus, diabetes mellitus, adrenal insufficiency)

- Malignancy

- Neurological (cerebral palsy, central nervous system tumors, neuromuscular or neurodegenerative disorders)

- Collagen vascular disorder

- Primary immunodeficiency

- Transplantation

- Adenoid/ tonsillar hypertrophy

- Inborn error of metabolism (Organic acidosis, storage disease)

- Sickle cell disease

PATHOGENESIS OF GROWTH RETARDATION IN ATOPIC DERMATITIS

One of the complications associated with atopic dermatitis is growth impairment in affected children, which may be attributed to following factors:[1, 9, 58]

- Decreased nocturnal growth hormone release

- Dysregulation of prostaglandin E2

- Hypoproteinemia

- Food allergy and unnecessary dietary restriction

- Coexisting asthma

- Corticosteroid therapy

- Severity of disease

Decreased Nocturnal Growth Hormone Release

GH is secreted from anterior pituitary. It is a major determinant of growth and metabolism and mediates its effects on target cells primarily by IGF-I, that is secreted from the liver and other tissues in response to growth hormone. IGF-I acts via activation of the IGF-I receptor. This receptor is widely distributed, which enables it to coordinate balanced growth among multiple tissues and organs, stimulating proliferation and differentiation of chondrocytes, myoblasts and protein synthesis. Deficiency in GH or defects in its binding to receptor are clinically manifested by growth retardation or dwarfism.[59-62]

Secretion of GH is affected by many factors, including stress, exercise, nutrition and sleep. Growth hormone secretion is also controlled by various hormones, such as growth hormone-releasing hormone (GHRH), a hypothalamic peptide and ghrelin from the stomach, stimulates its secretion, while somatostatin inhibits growth hormone release. GH is mainly secreted at night, shortly after the onset of deep sleep.[59, 63]

Sleep is an important physiological process, which is regulated by various cytokines and hormones. Altered sleep can also in turn affect their expression. GHRH promotes non-rapid eye movement sleep, while ghrelin and pro-inflammatory cytokines, such as IL-1 and TNF-α increase slow wave sleep and anti-inflammatory cytokines, such as IL-4 and IL-10 inhibit sleep.[59, 64] Sleep deprivation also tends to alter various cytokines expression, as loss of sleep decreases the nocturnal IL-6, which is a potent stimulator of hypothalamic pituitary axis, causing adrenocorticotrophic hormone (ACTH), cortisol and GH release.[65, 66] As it is hard for atopic dermatitis children to have a deep sleep since they frequently wake up at night to itch[67, 68], they are unable to release GH after falling asleep.[69,70] Ghrelin levels are also affected by sleep deprivation in atopics, so resulting in impaired growth hormone release.[71]

The release of growth hormone and its effects may also be influenced by poor nutrition. Fibroblast growth factor 21 (FGF21), a hormone induced by fasting, causes GH resistance. FGF21 decreases the formation of the active form of signal transducer and activator of transcription 5 (STAT5) in liver, which is a major mediator of GH actions, and causes corresponding reduction in the expression of its target genes, including insulin-like growth factor 1 (IGF-1), and results in growth stunting. Patients with atopic dermatitis may have food allergy or on unnecessary dietary restriction, which may result in poor nutrition and growth impairment.[72]

The secretion of GH is also affected by stress, and atopic patients are known to suffer from psychological stress due to their disease, which can impair growth of child.[1, 60]

Dysregulation of Prostaglandin E2

Atopy related imbalance in local growth factors like prostaglandin E2 (PGE_2), which is a substance important for both allergic reactions and bone metabolism, can also be a factor responsible for growth failure in children with atopic dermatitis. Prostaglandins are important regulators of bone metabolism. They stimulate bone remodeling, which depends on the target cell population, concentration of PGE_2 and its receptors. It might have an inhibitory effect on bone metabolism under pathological conditions when PGE_2 is present in high concentrations and for long periods[73]. The secretion of PGE_2 is increased in AD due to persistent macrophages activation, the resulting abnormality in the production of PGE_2 in atopics, may impair growth of child.[9, 22]

Hypoproteinemia

Children suffering from extensive AD fail to thrive, because of hypoalbuminaemia. Severity of disease is a risk factor for hypoproteinemia in AD, as large amounts of protein rich exudate is lost through the skin, at a rate that outstrips the synthesis of proteins. Food allergy can also result in decrease dietary intake and loss through gastrointestinal tract, resulting in hypoproteinemia.[74, 75]

Food Allergy and Unnecessary Dietary Restriction

Atopic patients may have allergy to certain foods, which may aggravate their disease. The prevalence of food allergy in patients with atopic dermatitis varies with the age of the patient, as it is more common in younger children than in older children and adults.[1] Dairy products, beef, eggs, chicken, fish, wheat, citrus fruits, food additives, chocolate and nuts, vasodilatory agents, such as alcohol, spices, and hot drinks, histamine-containing foods such as cheeses, very ripe vegetables such as tomatoes are common food allergens. Food allergy can be confirmed by food challenge test or by measuring specific IgE or prick testing. If there is a clearly identified aggravating factor in food, elimination of relevant dietary agent can lead to improvement in skin symptoms, but unnecessary dietary restrictions may cause malnutrition and growth failure in child.[1, 14]

Coexisting Asthma

Other allergic disorders of atopic diathesis such as asthma and allergic rhinitis, are also found to impair growth due to change in local growth factors PGE2 and IGF-1. So coexisting asthma or allergic rhinitis may further increase the risk of growth failure. Early onset, duration and severity of disease, hypoxemia, chronic anorexia and use of corticosteroids may be the precipitating factors for growth retardation in asthmatics.[76]

Corticosteroids

Growth impairment is a side effect of high-dose glucocorticoid therapy in childhood, when given in supraphysiological doses. Corticosteroids impair release of growth hormone and decreased activity of IGF-1 in growing bones. In proliferative chondrocytes, GH, parathyroid hormone (PTH) and 1, 25-dihydroxyvitamin D [1α, $25(OH)_2$ D_3] stimulates growth through secretion of IGF-I. Corticosteroids decrease GH, PTH or 1α, $25(OH)_2$ D_3 stimulated cells growth by reducing basal and hormone-stimulated IGF-I secretion. It also reduces levels of GH and the expression of the GH and IGF- I receptors.[77, 78]

Severity of Disease

Growth impairment in atopic dermatitis can be associated with severity of the disease. The more severe the disease, all the above discussed pathogenic factors would be accelerated, resulting in stunting of growth.[1]

ASSESSMENT OF GROWTH

The most powerful tool in growth assessment is the growth charts used in combination with accurate measurements of height, weight and head circumference, and by comparing an individual child's measurements with that of a large population with similar genetic background. Various growth charts have been developed after several studies to assess growth of children in United States, England and Sweden, but growth reference charts have yet to be developed in Pakistan for anthropometric measurement of our children, and National Centre of Health Statistics (NCHS) centile charts, published by the Centers for Disease Control and Prevention (CDC) of USA, are being used here.[79]

Measurements of patients are first taken and these measurements are plotted on 5 gender specific charts, as:

- Weight for age

- Height (length and stature) for age

- Head circumference for age

- Weight for height (length and stature)

- Body mass index (BMI) for children over 2 years of age

These charts have lines between 3rd /5th and 97th percentiles. These percentile curves indicate the percentage of children at a given age on x-axis whose measurements falls below the corresponding value on y-axis. The 50th percentile chart represents the median (standard value). Growth impairment refers to growth below the 3rd or 5th percentile or change in growth that has crossed two major growth percentiles in a short period of time.[52, 80]

MANAGEMENT AND PREVENTION OF GROWTH RETARDATION IN ATOPIC DERMATITIS

Regular growth assessment should be part of management of atopic dermatitis patients. It is important to identify the underlying precipitating factor of growth retardation, so as to undertake appropriate steps to improve health of a child. Severely affected child should be treated promptly. Steroids should be used with caution if child is already suffering from growth retardation and alternatives such as tacrolimus can be used.[15] Unnecessary dietary restrictions should be avoided; any associated asthma or allergic rhinitis should be managed accordingly.

OBJECTIVE

The objective of this study was to:

To determine the frequency of growth retardation in children with moderate to severe atopic dermatitis.

OPERATIONAL DEFINITIONS

ATOPIC DERMATITIS

The UK refinement of Hanifin and Rajka's diagnostic criteria[1] was used for diagnosing atopic dermatitis patients. annexure 1

SEVERITY

Severity of disease was measured by using objective SCORAD index[81] (SCORing Atopic Dermatitis) annexure 2

On the basis of SCORAD score, severity of atopic dermatitis was classified as;

Moderate = 15-40

Severe = >40

GROWTH RETARDATION

Growth retardation was assessed by using weight and height percentiles of National Centre of Health Statistics (NCHS), USA, by using weight for age, length / stature for age, weight for length / stature charts. Boys and girls with length / stature for age, weight for age or weight for length / stature less than 3rd percentile were taken as suffering from growth retardation.[82]

MATERIAL AND METHODS

SETTING

WAPDA Hospital, Lahore, a 300 bedded facility.

DURATION OF STUDY

Six months starting from March 2015 - August 2015

SAMPLE SIZE

The calculated sample size was 40 cases with 15% margin of error, 95% confidence level, taking expected percentage of children who had height below 3rd percentile (growth retardation) i.e. 34%.

SAMPLING TECHNIQUE

Non-probability purposive sampling

STUDY DESIGN

Cross sectional survey

SAMPLE SELECTION

Inclusion Criteria

- One to fifteen years of age

- Either sex

- Moderate to severe atopic dermatitis as mentioned operationary

Exclusion Criteria

- History of co-existing itchy skin disease e.g. Scabies

- History of systemic steroids intake for greater than 4 months at one time

- Any systemic disease which can cause growth retardation e.g. Asthma, congenital heart disease, rickets etc

- Mild atopic dermatitis with SCORAD score < 15

DATA COLLECTION

Forty children with atopic dermatitis fulfilling the inclusion criteria were entered in the study. After taking informed consent from parents, demographic information was recorded. Height was recorded, in centimeters, using infantometer in children ≤ 3 years of age and with stadiometer in patients > 3 years. Weight was taken, in kilograms, using Tanita baby scale for children ≤ 3 years of age and Bath room weighing scale for patients > 3 years. Growth charts were selected according to age and gender of patient, as when measuring boys and girls, 3 years and less than 3 years of age in recumbent position; length for age, weight for age and weight for length charts were used and for boys and girls > 3 years of age; weight for age, stature for age and weight for stature charts were used. On appropriate chart, measurements were recorded, as patient's age on horizontal axis and by using a ruler a vertical line was drawn up from that point and measurements (length, stature, weight) were recorded on vertical axis and a horizontal line was drawn across that point until it intersect the vertical line and a small dot was marked where two lines intersect, if plotted dot was below 3rd percentile on any of these charts, then child was taken as suffering from growth retardation. Effect modifier like moderate and severe AD were addressed through stratification.

DATA ANALYSIS

All the data was entered and analyzed through SPSS (version 13.0). Age, weight and height of the children were presented by calculating mean ± standard deviation and frequency & percentage was calculated for gender and growth of child (normal, retarded). Data was stratified for moderate and severe atopic dermatitis to address the effect modifiers.

FREQUENCY OF GROWTH RETARDATION IN CHILDREN WITH MODERATE TO SEVERE ATOPIC DERMATITIS

PROFORMA

Case No_____OPD NO _____ Date_____

Name_____ D/O, S/O _____ Sex_____

Date of birth Day____ Month____ Year_____ Age_____

Weight (kg)_____ Height/length (cm) _____

Severity of atopic dermatitis Moderate □

Severe □

Growth assessment according to growth charts:

Weight for age percentiles

Less than 3rd percentile for age □

Between 3rd to 97th percentiles & above for age □

Length / Stature for age percentiles

Less than 3rd percentile for age □

Between 3rd to 97th percentiles & above for age □

Weight for Length / Stature percentiles

Less than 3rd percentile for age □

Between 3rd to 97th percentiles & above for age □

Conclusion

Growth of child Normal □

Retarded □

RESULTS

Forty children, 21 (52.5%) male and 19 (47.5%) female, age ranging from 1 to 14.10 years (mean age 5.86 ± 4.01 years), suffering from moderate to severe atopic dermatitis were enrolled in the study (Table 1, Fig 1, 2).

Mean height and weight, with standard deviation (SD) of these children are shown in Fig 3 and 4. When the weight and height of the patients were plotted on NCHS growth charts for their respective age and sex, 25 (62.5%) children had normal growth while 15 (37.5%) patients had retarded growth (Fig 5). Among these 15 children, 9 (22.5%) were suffering from severe disease and 6 (15%) had moderate disease. Out of 40 patients, 11 had severe disease and 6 (54.54%) of them were suffering from growth retardation, while 29 had moderate disease and 9 (31.03%) of them showed impaired growth (Fig 6). Nine (22.5%) of the patients with growth impairment were female and 6 (15%) were male (Fig 7).

Table 1: Demographic Data

No. of Patients 40	
Male	21
Female	19
Age (mean)	5.86 ±4.01years
Minimum	1year
Maximum	14.10 years

FIGURE I

Age distribution

(n= 40)

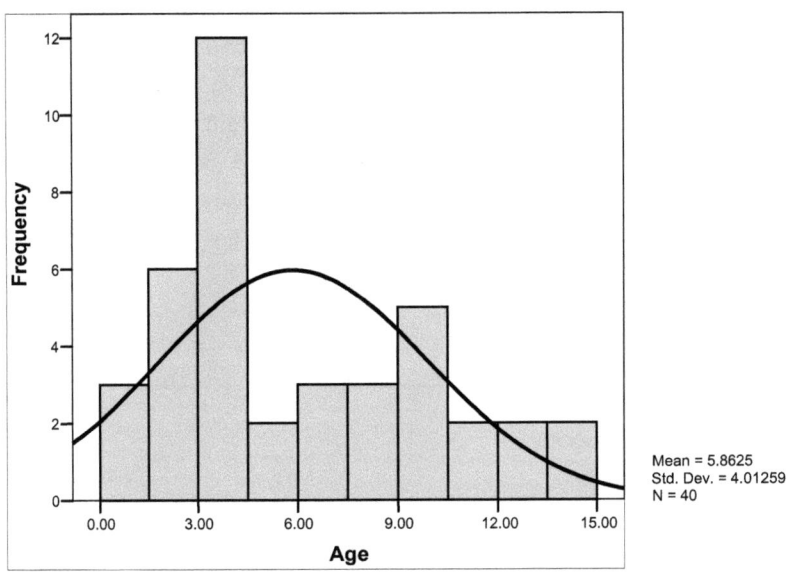

FIGURE II

Sex distribution

(n= 40)

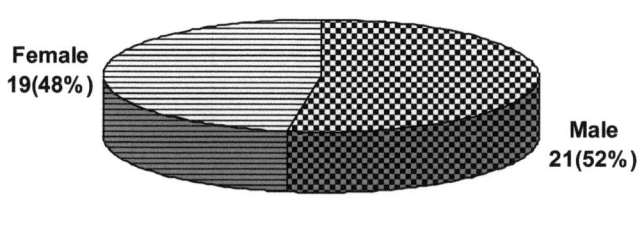

Figure III

Height distribution

(n= 40)

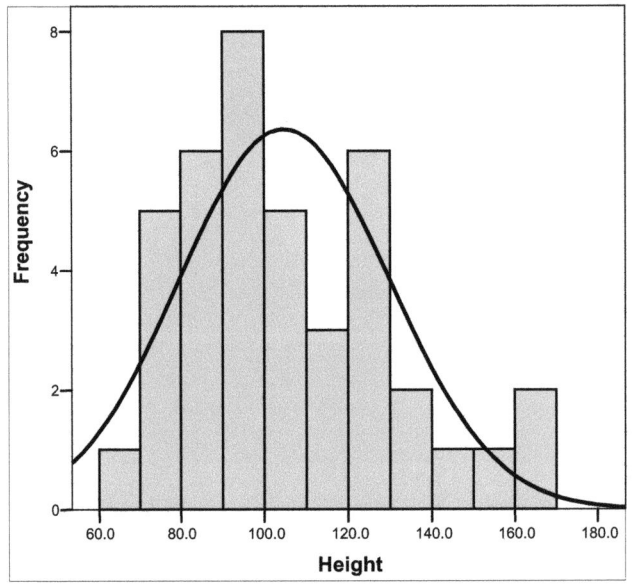

Mean = 104.725
Std. Dev. = 25.0712
N = 40

FIGURE IV

Weight distribution

(n= 40)

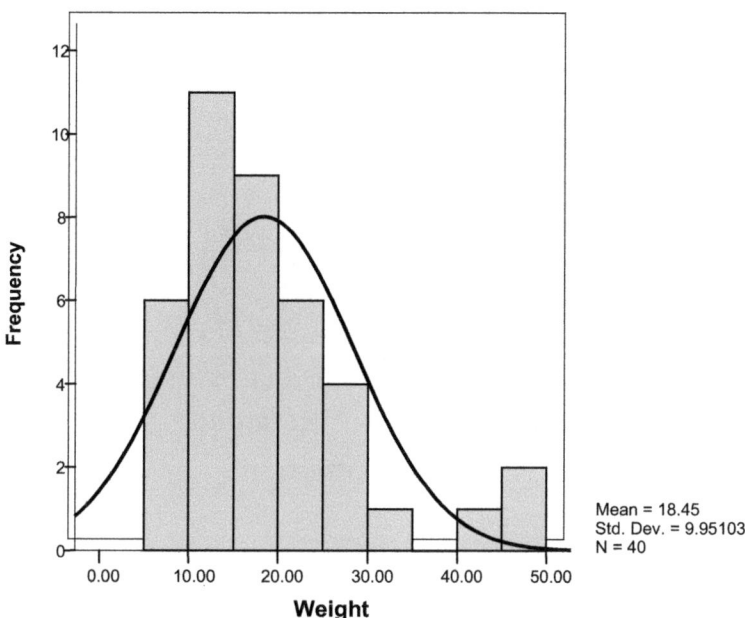

FIGURE V

Comparison of normal

&

growth retarded children

(n=40)

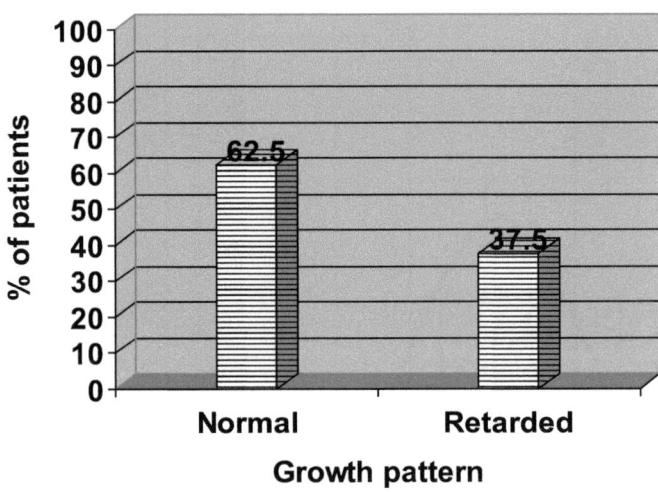

FIGURE VI

Comparison of growth between moderate and severe Atopic
Dermatitis

(n= 40)

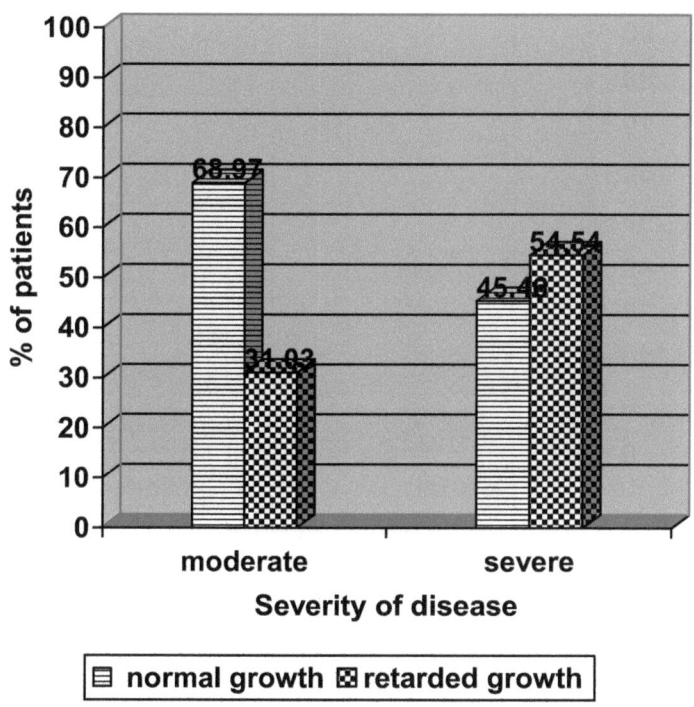

FIGURE VII

Comparison of growth retardation in male and female
(n=40)

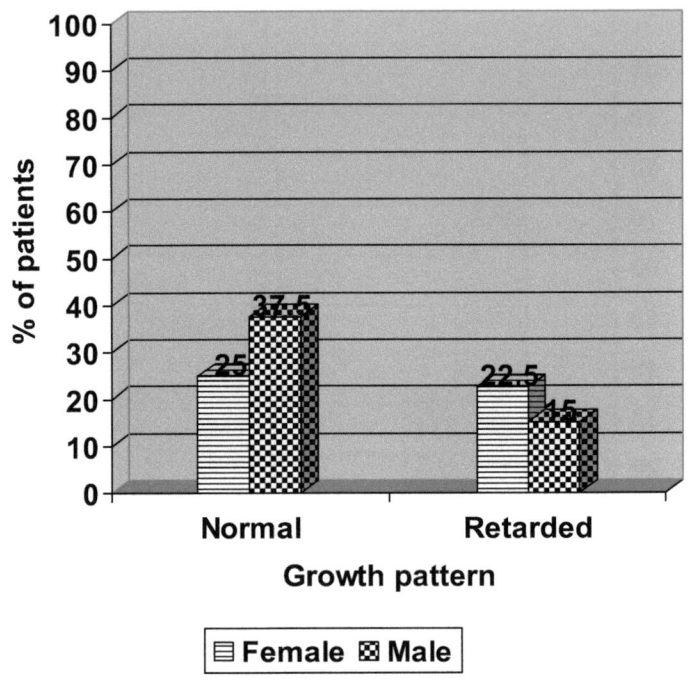

DISCUSSION

Atopic dermatitis has profound impact on quality of life and causes significant morbidity. One of the complications associated with atopic dermatitis is growth impairment in affected children. In this study, we found impaired growth in 37.5% of children suffering from moderate to severe atopic dermatitis. Our observations are supported by other studies, as Kristmundsdottir et al. reported retarded growth in 10% of his patients.[83] Similar study at the Department of Child Health, University of Manchester, England found that short stature was present in 22% of children with atopic eczema.[84]

A positive association was seen to exist between the occurrence of growth retardation in children with atopic dermatitis and the severity of the disease and also with the surface area of involvement in present study. Our results are compatible with other studies, as Massarano et al.[13] and Myoshi et al.[85] also found that growth of the patients was significantly affected by the severity of the disease. Multiple factors may be involved in causing growth retardation in children suffering from severe atopic dermatitis. More aggressive treatment in form of potent topical steroids or oral steroids for disease control can have effect on growth. Systemic steroids and/or potent topical steroids might have been misused in our patients in severe disease, before presenting to us. Atopic children also have poor sleep due to pruritus, which impairs release of nocturnal growth hormone. Growth retardation in these severely affected patients may also be due to loss of proteins through skin and gastrointestinal tract, leading to hypoproteinemia. In our community, unnecessary dietary restrictions due to fear of food allergy are often self imposed or even encouraged by quacks, hakeems and relatives in desperate attempts or false beliefs to get relief of a chronic disease like atopic dermatitis, which has a great impact on quality of life. In developing country like ours, caring for patients with some chronic disease, may also impose a high economic burden on the family, leading to child neglect and malnourishment.

The frequency of growth retardation was more in female patients in the present study. This association between growth impairment and sex of the patients is important, as in many previous studies, growth of boys and girls were not evaluated separately, and only a few have analyzed sex difference. Palit et al. in a study in India found that girls, aged 3-5 years with AD had poor growth than boys[8]. In our study, the growth pattern of affected child and sex was similar to this Indian study. The number of female patients with severe disease were more in Palit et al. study, while in our study there was no significant difference in severity of disease in males and females. The cause of this gender difference seems to be the interplay of different physiological, environmental, socioeconomic and cultural factors. The preferential care and treatment given to male children in contrast to females in existing subcontinent culture, could contribute to this difference. The objective of this study was to highlight the importance of regular growth monitoring in children with AD, who may be at greater risk of suffering from impaired growth due to disease process itself and also the treatment given to them, in form of steroids, may further perpetuate this problem. More studies with a larger sample size can be carried out in Pakistan, to evaluate the growth pattern of patients suffering from this chronic disorder, its possible underlying factors and to demonstrate any impact of sex difference on growth in our children.

CONCLUSION

These results show growth retardation in children with atopic dermatitis and the frequency of growth impairment was relatively more in severe disease and among girls, as depicted by growth charts.

REFERENCES

1. Friedmann PS, Holden CA. Atopic dermatitis. In: Burns T, Breathnach S, Cox N, Griffiths C, editors. Rook's Textbook of Dermatology 7th ed. Blackwell science publication, London; 2004: 18.1-18.2.

2. Nasreen S, Wahid Z, Ahmed A. Atopic dermatitis: Frequency of associated disorders in children. J Pak Assoc Dermatol 2005; 15: 125-9.

3. Ejaz A, Raza N. Management of atopic dermatitis, A review. J Pak Assoc Dermatol 2004; 14: 140-7.

4. Leung DY, Bieber T. Atopic dermatitis. Lancet 2003; 361: 151-60.

5. Brown S, Reynolds NJ. Atopic and non- atopic eczema. BMJ 2006; 332: 584-8.

6. Ahmed I, Ansari M, Malick K. Childhood eczema: a comparative analysis. J Pak Assoc Dermatol 2003; 13: 164-70.

7. William HC. Atopic dermatitis. N Eng J Med 2005; 352: 2314-24.

8. Palit A, Handa S, Bhalla AK, Kumar B. A mixed longitudinal study of physical growth in children with atopic dermatitis. Ind J Dermatol Venereol Leprol 2007; 73: 171-5.

9. Baum WF, Schneyer U, Lantzsch AM, Kloditz E. Delay of growth and development in children with bronchial asthma, atopic dermatitis and allergic rhinitis. Exp Clin Endocrinol Diabetes 2002; 110: 53-9.

10. David TJ, Ferguson AP, Newton RW. Nocturnal growth hormone release in children with short stature and atopic dermatitis. Acta Derm venereol 1991; 71: 229-31.

11. Deshmukh CT. Minimizing side effects of systemic corticosteroids in children. Ind J Dermatol Venereol Leprol 2007; 73: 218-21.

12. Dhar S, Mondal B, Malakar R, Ghosh A, Gupta AB. Correlation of severity of atopic dermatitis with growth retardation in pediatric age group. Ind J Dermatol 2005; 50: 125-8.

13. Massarano AA, Hollis S, Devlin J, David TJ. Growth in atopic eczema. Arch Dis Child 1993; 68: 677-9.

14. Atopic Dermatitis. [Cited 2009 May 22]. Available from: http: / /www Dermatology online journal.

15. Bieber T. Atopic Dermatitis. N Eng J Med 2008; 358: 1483-94.

16. Wadonda NK, Sterne JA, Golding J, Kennedy CT, Archer CB, Dunnill MG. A prospective study of the prevalence and incidence of atopic dermatitis in children aged 0-42 months. Br J Dermatol 2003; 149: 1023-8.

17. Leung DY, Boguniewicz M, Howell MD, Nomura I, Hamid QA. New insights into atopic dermatitis. J Clin Invest 2004; 113: 651-57.

18. Leung DY, Eichenfield LF, Boguniewicz M. Atopic dermatitis. In: Wolff K, Goldsmith LA, Katz SI, Gilchrest BA, Paller AS, Leffel DJ. Fitzpatrick's dermatology in general medicine 6th ed. McGraw-Hill, New York; 2003: 146- 58.

19. James WD, Berger TC, Elston DM. Andrew's diseases of the skin: Clinical dermatology 10th ed. Saunders Elsevier publications, Canada; 2000: 69-76.

20. Cantani A. Pathogenesis of atopic dermatitis and the role of allergic factors. Eur Rev Med Pharmacol Sci 2001; 5: 95-117.

21. Neaville WA, Tisler C, Bhattacharya A, Anklam K, White GS, Hamilton R et al. Developmental cytokine response profiles and the clinical and immunologic expression of atopy during the first year of life. J Allergy Clin Immunol 2003; 112: 740–6.

22. Giménez JC. Atopic dermatitis: Review article. Alergol Inmunol Clin 2000; 15: 279-95.

23. McGirt LY, Beck LA. Innate immune defects in atopic dermatitis. J Allergy Clin Immunol 2006; 118: 202-8.

24. Stemmler S, Parwez Q, Parwez EP, Epplen JT, Hoffjan S. Two common loss-of-function mutations within the filaggrin gene predispose for early onset of atopic dermatitis. J Invest Dermatol 2007; 127: 722–24.

25. Blyumin ML, Hu S and Kirsner RS. Filaggrin Gene Mutations Mediate Severity of Alopecia Areata When Associated with Atopic Dermatitis. J Invest Dermatol 2007; 127: 2494.

26. Sandilands A, O'Regan GM, Liao H, Zhao Y, Kwiatkowski AT, Watson RM et al. Prevalent and rare mutations in the gene encoding filaggrin cause ichthyosis vulgaris and predispose individuals to atopic dermatitis. J Invest Dermatol 2006; 126: 1770–75.

27. Weidinger S, Illig T, Baurecht H, Irvine AD, Rodriguez E, Lacava DA et al. Loss-of-function variations within the filaggrin gene predispose for atopic dermatitis with allergic sensitizations. J Allergy Clin Immunol 2006; 118: 214-9.

28. Irvine AD, McLean WH. Breaking the unsound barrier: filaggrin is a major gene for atopic dermatitis. J Invest Dermatol 2006; 126: 1200-2.

29. Choi MJ, Maibach HI. Role of ceramides in barrier function of healthy and diseased skin. Am J Clin Dermatol 2005; 6: 215-23.

30. Cork MJ, Robinson DA, Vasilopoulos Y, Ferguson A, Moustafa M, MacGowan A et al. New perspective on epidermal barrier dysfunction in atopic dermatitis: gene-environment interaction. J Allergy Clin Immunol 2006; 118: 3-21.

31. Ong PY, Ohtake T, Brandt C, Strickland I, Boguniewicz M, Ganz T et al. Endogenous antimicrobial peptides and skin infections in atopic dermatitis. N End J Med 2002; 347: 1151-60.

32. Rieg S, Steffen H, Seeber S, Humeny A, Kalbacher H, Dietz K et al. Deficiency of dermcidin-derived antimicrobial peptides in sweat of patients with atopic dermatitis correlates with an impaired innate defense of human skin in vivo. J Immunol 2005; 174: 8003-10.

33. Arikawa J, Ishibashi M, Kawashima M, Takagi Y, Ichikawa Y, Imokawa G. Decreased levels of sphingosine, a natural antimicrobial agent, may be associated with vulnerability of the stratum corneum from patients with atopic dermatitis to colonization by Staphylococcus aureus. J Invest Dermatol 2002; 119: 433-9.

34. Benedetto AD, Agnihothri R, McGirt LY, Bankova LG, Beck LA. Atopic dermatitis: A disease caused by innate immune defects? J Invest Dermatol 2008; 129: 14-30.

35. Bloomfield SF, Smith RS, Crevel RW, Pickup J. Too clean, or not too clean: the hygiene hypothesis. J Clin Exp Allergy 2006; 36: 402-25.

36. Von Mutius E, Fahrländer BC, Schierl R, Riedler J, Ehlermann S, Maisch S et al. Exposure to endotoxin or other bacterial components might protect against the development of atopy. Clin Exp Allerg 2000; 30: 1230-34.

37. Sherriff A, Golding J. Hygiene levels in a contemporary population cohort are associated with wheezing and atopic eczema in preschool infants. Arch Dis Child 2002; 87: 26-9.

38. Kilpi T, Kero J, J Jokinen, Syrjanen R, Takala AK, Hovi T et al . Common respiratory infections early in life may reduce the risk of atopic dermatitis. Clin Infect Dis 2002; 34: 620-26.

39. Hon KL, Lam MC, Wong KY, Leung TF, Ng PC. Pathophysiology of nocturnal scratching in childhood atopic dermatitis: the role of brain-derived neurotrophic factor and substance P. Br J Dermatol 2007; 157: 922-5.

40. Kaujalgi R, Handa S, Jain A, Kanwar AJ. Ocular abnormalities in atopic dermatitis in Indian patients. Ind J Dermatol Venerol 2009; 75: 148-51.

41. Carmi E, Tribout CD, Ganry O, Cene S, Tramier B, Milazzo S et al. Ocular complications of atopic dermatitis in children. Acta Derm Venereol 2006; 86: 515-17.

42. Hayashi H, Igarashi C, Hayashi K. Frequency of ciliary body or retinal breaks and retinal detachment in eyes with atopic cataract. Br J Ophthamol 2002; 86: 898-901.

43. Andrew Tatham. Atopic dermatitis, cutaneous steroids and cataracts in children: two case reports. J Med Case Reports 2008; 2: 124.

44. Manjunath S, Suchitra U. Kaposi's varicelliform eruption. Ind J Dermatol Venerol 2007; 73: 65.

45. Peng WM, Jenneck C, Bussmann C, Bagdanow M, Hart J, Leung DY et al. Risk factors of atopic dermatitis patients for eczema herpeticum. J Invest Dermatol 2007; 127: 1261-63.

46. Watanabe S, Kano R, Sato H, Nakamura Y, Hasegawa A. The effects of Malassezia yeasts on cytokine production by human keratinocytes. J Invest Dermatol 2001; 116: 769-73.

47. Scheynius A, Johansson C, Buentke E, Zargari A, Linder MT. Atopic eczema/dermatitis syndrome and Malassezia. Int Arch Allergy Immunol 2002; 127: 161-9.

48. Roll A, Cozzio A, Fischer B, Peter SG. Microbial colonization and atopic dermatitis. Curr Opin Allergy Clin Immunol 2004; 4: 373–78.

49. Lin YT, Wang CT, Hsu CT, Wang LF, Shau WY, Yang YH et al. Differential susceptibility to staphylococcal superantigen (SsAg)-induced apoptosis of CD4+ T cells from atopic dermatitis patients and healthy subjects: the inhibitory effect of IL-4 on SsAg-induced apoptosis. J Immunol 2003; 171: 1102-8.

50. Lissaurer T, Clayden G. Illustrated text book of paedriatrics 3rd ed. Mosby Elsevier publications, London; 2008: 169-97.

51. Edouard T, Trivin CE, Body EL, Pinto G, Souberbielle JC, Brauner R. Extreme short stature after intrauterine growth retardation: Factors associated with lack of catch-up growth. Horm Res 2004; 61: 33-40.

52. Bauchner H. Failure to thrive. In: Behrman K, Stantan J, editors. Nelson textbook of paedriatrics18th ed. Elsevier publications. 2009:184-87.

53. Venkateshwar V, Raman TR. Failure to thrive: Review article. Mjafi 2000; 56: 219-24.

54. Sultan M, Afzal M, Qureshi SM, Aziz S, Lutfullah M, Khan SA et al. Etiology of short stature in children. J Coll Physicians Surg Pak 2008; 18: 493-97.

55. Block RW, Krebs NF. Failure to Thrive as a Manifestation of Child Neglect. Pediatrics 2005; 116: 1234-37.

56. Miller TL, Easley KA, Zhang W, Orav EJ, Bier DM, Luder E et al. Maternal and infant factors associated with failure to thrive in children with vertically transmitted human immunodeficiency virus-1 infection: The prospective, P^2C^2 Human immunodeficiency virus multicenter study. Pediatrics 2001; 108: 1287-96.

57. The European collaborative study. Height, weight, and growth in children born to mothers with HIV-1 infection in Europe. Pediatrics 2003; 111: 52-60.

58. Agostoni C, Grandi F, Scaglioni S, Giannì ML, Torcoletti M, Radaelli G et al. Growth pattern of breastfed and nonbreastfed infants with atopic dermatitis in the first year of life. Pediatrics 2000; 106: 73.

59. McDowall J. Growth hormone receptor. [Cited on 2009 May 29] Available on: www.ebi.ac.uk/interpro/potm/2004_4/Page1.htm

60. Rosenbloom AL. Physiology of Growth. Ann Nestlé Engl 2007; 65: 97-108.

61. Butler AA, Le Roith D. Control of growth by the somatropic axis: growth hormone and the insulin-like growth factors have related and independent roles. Annu Rev Physiol 2001; 63: 141-64.

62. Woelfle J, Chia DJ, Rotwein P. Mechanism of growth hormone action. Identification of conserved Stat5 binding sites that mediates GH-induced insulin-like growth factor-1 gene activation. J Biol Chem 2003; 278: 51261-6.

63. Growth hormone. [Cited on 2009 june 15] Available on: http://www.colostate.edu/hbooks/pathphys/endocrine/hypopit/gh.html

64. Majde JA, Krueger JM. Links between the innate immune system and sleep. J Allergy Clin Immunol 2005; 116: 1188-98.

65. Schwalbe ES, Hansen K, Schmidt F, Schrezenmeier H, Marshall L, Burger K. Acute effects of recombinant human interleukin-6 on endocrine and central nervous sleep functions in healthy men. J Clin Endocrinol Metabol 1998; 83: 1573-79.

66. Redwine L, Hauger RL, Gillin JC, Irwin M. Effects of sleep and sleep deprivation on interleukin-6, growth hormone, cortisol, and melatonin levels in humans. J Clin Endocrinol & Metabol 2000; 85: 3597-3603.

67. Beattie PE, Jones ML. An audit of the impact of a consultation with a paediatric dermatology team on quality of life in infants with atopic eczema and their families. Br J Dermatol 2006; 155:1249-55.

68. Bender BG, Leung SB, Leung DY. Actigraphy assessment of sleep disturbance in patients with atopic dermatitis: An objective life quality measure. J Allergy Clin Immunol 2003; 111: 598-602.

69. Cauter EV. Inadequate sleep affects hormone levels. J Am Med Assoc 2000; 284: 861-81.

70. Bendert BG, Leung DM. Sleep disorders in patients with asthma, atopic dermatitis, and allergic rhinitis. J Allergy Clin Immunol 2005; 116: 1200-01.

71. Kimata H. Viewing humorous film improves night-time wakening in children with atopic dermatitis. Ind Pedriatrics 2007; 44: 281-84.

72. Inagaki T, Lin VY , Goetz R, Mohammadi M, Mangelsdor DJ, Kliewer SA. Inhibition of growth hormone signaling by fasting induced hormones FGF21. Cell Metabolism 2008; 8: 77-83.

73. Samoto H, Shimizu E, Honjyo YM, Saito R, Nakao S, Yamazaki M. Prostaglandin E_2 stimulates bone sialoprotein (BSP) expression through cAMP and fibroblast growth factor 2 response elements in the proximal promoter of the rat BSP gene. J Biol Chem 2003; 278: 28659-67.

74. Nomura I, Katsunuma T, Tomikawa M, Shibata A, Kawahara H, Ohya Y et al. Hypoproteinemia in severe childhood atopic dermatitis: A serious complication. Ped Allergy Immunol 2008; 13: 287-94.

75. Katoh N, Hosoi H, SugimotoT, Kishimoto S. Features and prognoses of infantile patients with atopic dermatitis hospitalized for severe complications. J Dermatol 2006; 33: 827-32.

76. Antonio MA, Ribeiro JD, Toro AA, Piedrabuena AE, Morcillo AM. Linear growth in asthmatic children. J Pneumol 2003; 29: 36-42.

77. Klaus G, Jux C, Fernandez P, Rodriguez J, Himmele R, Mehls O. Suppression of growth plate chondrocytes proliferation by corticosteroids. Pediatr Nephrol 2000; 14: 612-14.

78. Lai HC, Fitz SC, Allen DB. Risk of persistent growth impairment after alternate-day prednisone treatment in children with cystic fibrosis. N Eng J Med. 2000; 342: 851–59.

79. Aziz S, Puri DA, Hussain KZ, Hussain F, Naqvi SA, Rizvi SA. Anthropometric indices of middle socioeconomic class school children in Karachi compared with NCHS standards- A pilot study. J Pak Med Assoc 2006; 56: 264.

80. Keane V. Assessment of growth. In: Behrman K, Stantan J, editors. Nelson textbook of paedriatrics18th ed. Elsevier publications. 2009: 70-74.

81. Oranje AP, Glazenburg EJ, Wolkerstorfer A, Waard-van FB. Practical issues on interpretation of scoring atopic dermatitis: the SCORAD index, objective SCORAD and the three-item severity score. Br J Dermatol 2007; 157: 645-8.

82. NCHS – 2000 CDC Growth Charts: United States. [Cited 2008 May 2]. Available from: http: / /www.cdc.gov/ GROWTH CHARTS.

83. Kristmundsdottir F, David TJ. Growth impairment in children with atopic eczema. J R Soc Med 1987; 80: 9-12.

84. David TJ. Short stature in children with atopic eczema. Acta Derm Venerol Suppl 1989; 144: 41-4.

85. Miyoshi M, Sakurai T, Kodama S. Growth impairment in infants with atopic dermatitis. Arerugi 1996; 45: 41-8.

Annexure 1

The child must have an itchy skin condition (or parental report of scratching or rubbing in a child) plus 3 or more of following:

- Onset below 2 years (not used if child is under 4 years)

- History of skin crease involvement (and/or cheeks in children under 10 years)

- History of generally dry skin

- Personal history of other atopic disease (or history of any atopic disease in a first degree relative in children under 4 years)

- Visible flexural dermatitis (or dermatitis of cheeks/ forehead and outer limbs in children under 4 years)

Annexure 2

SCORAD INDEX is based on 2 sub score:

A) Extent score based on body surface area involved, using rule of nine.

B) Intensity score based on 6 clinical findings in atopic dermatitis which include erythema, oedema/papulation, excoriation, lichenification, oozing/crusts and dryness. Each finding has 4 scoring points ranging from 0 to 3; 0=absent ;1= mild; 2=moderate ; 3= severe

SCORAD INDEX=A/5+ 7B/2

Maximum SCORAD score is 83 (plus an additional 10 bonus points for severe eczema on face and hands)

YOUR KNOWLEDGE HAS VALUE

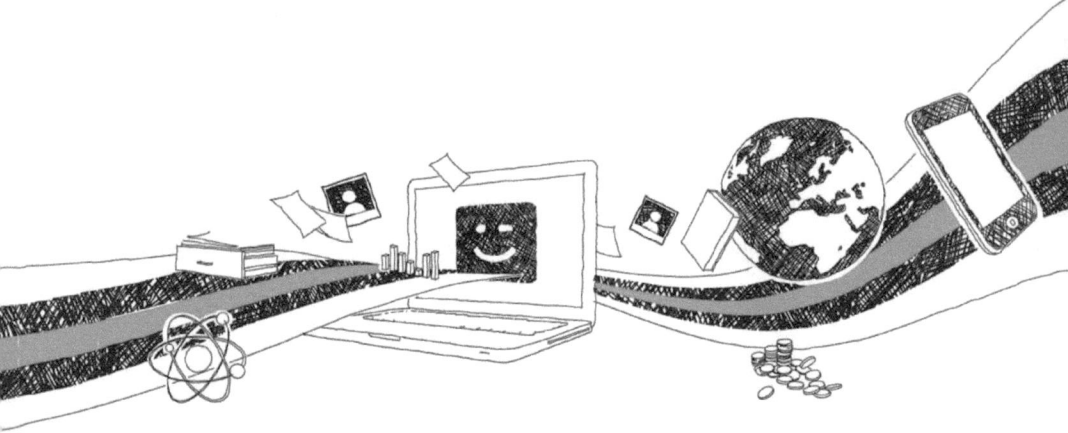

- We will publish your bachelor's and master's thesis, essays and papers

- Your own eBook and book - sold worldwide in all relevant shops

- Earn money with each sale

Upload your text at www.GRIN.com
and publish for free

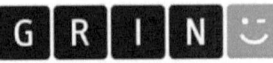